Your Daily Diary & Health Journal

Helping You Live Your Best Life

Basic Health
PUBLICATIONS, INC.

The information contained in this book is not intended as a substitute for consulting with your physician or other healthcare provider. Any attempt to diagnose and treat an illness should be done under the direction of a health care professional.

The publisher does not advocate the use of any particular healthcare protocol but believes the information in this book should be available to the public. The publisher is not responsible for any adverse effects or consequence resulting from the use of the suggestions, preparations, or procedures discussed in this book. Should the reader have any questions concerning the appropriateness of any procedures or preparation mentioned, the publisher strongly suggests consulting a professional healthcare advisor.

Basic Health Publications, Inc.
8200 Boulevard East
North Bergen, NJ 07047
1-201-868-8336

ISBN: 1-59120-144-6

Editor: Carol Rosenberg
Typesetting/Book design: Gary A. Rosenberg
Cover design: Mike Stromberg

Printed in the United States of America

10   9   8   7   6   5   4   3   2   1

This journal belongs to:

Address:

Phone number(s):

In case of an emergency, contact:

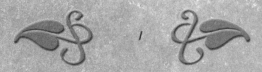

Blood type:

_____

Organ-donor preference:

_____

*Insurance carrier and
group or policy number(s):*

_____

_____

_____

Secondary insurance carrier:

_____

_____

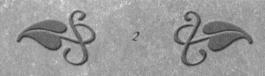

Doctors, dentists, and specialists:

_____

_____

_____

_____

_____

_____

_____

_____

_____

_____

_____

_____

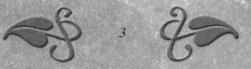

My pharmacy information:

_____

_____

_____

Medications and supplements
I am currently taking:

_____

_____

_____

_____

_____

_____

_____

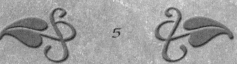

Medical problems I have had and when:

_____

_____

_____

_____

_____

_____

_____

_____

_____

_____

_____

_____

_____

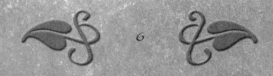

Operations or procedures I have had and when:

_____

_____

_____

_____

_____

_____

_____

_____

_____

_____

_____

_____

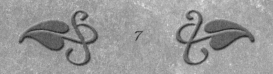

Family health history:

_____

_____

_____

_____

_____

_____

_____

_____

_____

_____

_____

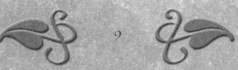

Dates to remember:

_____

_____

_____

_____

_____

_____

_____

_____

_____

_____

_____

_____

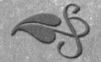 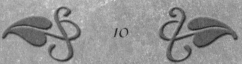

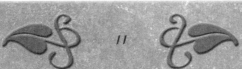

What is a weed?
A plant whose virtues
have not yet been discovered.
—RALPH WALDO EMERSON

Today's Date

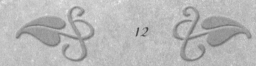

Many common herbs—from chamomile and garlic to turmeric and willowbark—have medicinal uses that you may find helpful in your quest for good health.

Today's Date

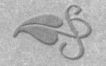

> Health is the thing that makes you
> feel that now is the best time of the year.
>
> —FRANKLIN P. ADAMS

Today's Date

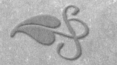

Good health promotes energy, confidence, productivity, and well-being. All of these factors can lead to a more fulfilling life.

Today's Date

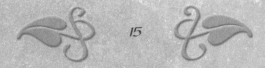

> Change is not made without
> inconvenience, even from worse to better.
> —RICHARD HOOKER

Today's Date

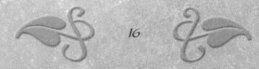

When making positive lifestyle changes,
it may be easier to make many small changes
a few at a time than to make a few major
changes all at once.

_____

Today's Date

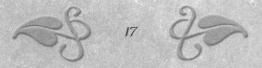

> A little health now and again
> is the ailing person's best remedy.
> —FRIEDRICH NIETZSCHE

Today's Date

Because they are usually gentler on the system, natural remedies often take longer to have a noticeable effect than their chemical counterparts.

Today's Date

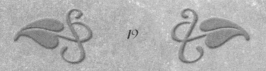

> Happiness consists in a
> frequent repetition of pleasure.
>
> —ARTHUR SCHOPENHAUER

Today's Date

Doing something you enjoy for at least
a half hour each evening can help you
decompress after a hard day's work
at the office or in the field.

Today's Date

> Despise no new accident
> in your body, but ask opinion of it.
> —FRANCIS BACON

_____

Today's Date

Periodically examine your skin from head to toe for any changes. Tell your doctor right away if you notice anything out of the ordinary.

Today's Date

> Find out for yourself
> the form of rest that refreshes you best.
> —DANIEL CONSIDINE

_____

Today's Date

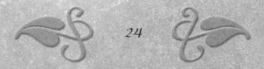

If you're having trouble sleeping, listen to soothing music in a quiet setting before turning in for the night. It may help you sleep more soundly.

Today's Date

> Eat breakfast like a king,
> lunch like a prince, and dinner like a pauper.
> —ADELLE DAVIS

Today's Date

Breakfast really *is* the most important meal of the day. A balanced breakfast is a great way to get your metabolism going. This will give you more energy throughout the day.

Today's Date

> Give me health and a day,
> and I will make the pomp of emperors ridiculous.
>
> —RALPH WALDO EMERSON

Today's Date

Reminding yourself of the things you are thankful for each morning may help put the rest of your day's events in the proper perspective.

Today's Date

> Health is a state of complete physical, mental and social well-being, and not merely the absence of disease or infirmity.
>
> —FROM THE CONSTITUTION OF THE WORLD HEALTH ORGANIZATION

Today's Date

The U.S. recommended daily allowances for vitamins and minerals were established to help prevent deficiency diseases. Higher doses may be needed for optimal health.

Today's Date

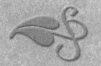

If you are visited by pain,
examine your conduct.
—Talmud

Today's Date

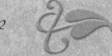

Injuries can occur as a result of repetitive movements or improper posture. Making adjustments to seating or workspace, and taking frequent short breaks, can help you avoid them.

Today's Date

> Moderation multiplies pleasures.
> —CLEOBULUS

Today's Date

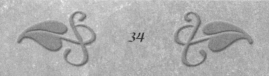

Sometimes even too much of a good thing can cause an imbalance in the body. Avoid exceeding what's suitable or required for your particular needs.

Today's Date

35

> The body never lies.
> —MARTHA GRAHAM

<u>Today's Date</u>

 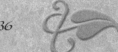

Listening to what your body has to say to you may be enlightening. It may be asking you to take better care of it—or it may just want to say "thank you!"

_____

Today's Date

37

> Laughter is the most healthful exertion.
> —Christoph Wilhelm Hufeland

Today's Date

Laughter has been shown to strengthen the immune system and decrease stress hormones. For good health, laugh as often as possible.

_____

Today's Date

_____
_____
_____
_____
_____
_____
_____
_____
_____
_____
_____
_____
_____
_____
_____

> Meditation and prayer are to the soul what reflection, study, and conversation are to the mind and what exercise, physical work, and sports are to the body.
>
> —Anonymous

Today's Date

~~~~~~~

_____

_____

_____

_____

_____

_____

_____

_____

_____

_____

_____

_____

_____

_____

_____

_____

_____

_____

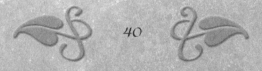

40

Regular practice of a meditation technique that you enjoy and that brings you a sense of peace can help reduce the stress of day-to-day living.

Today's Date

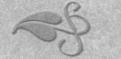

> It is more important to know
> what kind of patient has the disease than
> what kind of disease the patient has.
>
> —SIR WILLIAM OSLER

Today's Date

_____

_____

_____

_____

_____

_____

_____

_____

_____

_____

_____

_____

_____

_____

_____

_____

_____

_____

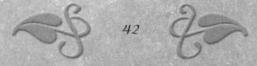

Many popular alternative forms of health care, such as homeopathy, focus on treating the whole person—not on suppressing the symptoms of the illness—to achieve good health.

Today's Date

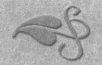

Take twice as long to eat half as much.

—ANONYMOUS

Today's Date

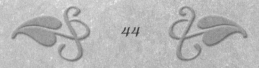

Rushing through meals can lead to unhealthy eating habits and digestive troubles. Eat slowly and mindfully, and engage in pleasant conversation.

_____

Today's Date

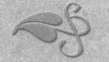

Never open the door to a
little vice lest a great one enter with it.
—Anonymous

Today's Date

Alcohol is a depressant, not a mood lifter.
It's wise to avoid drinking when you're alone
or if you're feeling down or depressed.

Today's Date

> Nothing in the world is
> difficult for one who sets his mind to it.
>
> —CHINESE SAYING

Today's Date

When trying to shed unwanted body fat,
a loss of one to two pounds per week is
generally considered to be a healthy goal.

Today's Date

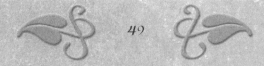

> Old age takes away from us what we
> have inherited and gives us what we have earned.
>
> —GERALD BRENAN

_____

Today's Date

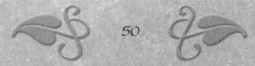

Regular exercise, a healthy diet,
and an optimistic outlook are essential
components of graceful aging.

Today's Date

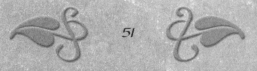

Health is the greatest gift, contentment
the greatest wealth, faithfulness the best relationship.
—Buddha

Today's Date

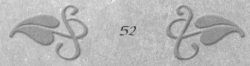

52

To improve your chances of maintaining your exercise routine, work out with a buddy. Exercise partners can support, encourage, and motivate each other.

Today's Date

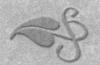

> Pain is part of the body's magic.
> It is the way the body transmits a sign to the brain
> that something is wrong.
> —NORMAN COUSINS

Today's Date

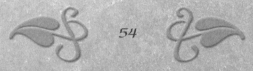

Masking your pain with over-the-counter pain relievers may bring temporary relief, but it's more important to identify the source of your pain and take steps to remedy it.

Today's Date

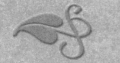

Sometimes your joy is the source
of your smile, but sometimes your smile
can be the source of your joy.

—THICH NHAT HANH

Today's Date

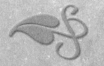

Anecdotal evidence suggests that the "placebo effect"—a benefit attributed to the belief that a substance or technique has worked—is sometimes just as effective as treatment.

Today's Date

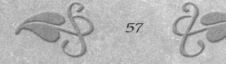

> The best and most beautiful things
> in the world cannot be seen or even touched.
> They must be felt with the heart.
> —HELEN KELLER

Today's Date

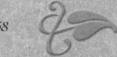

A wholesome diet low in cholesterol and saturated fats, as well as regular exercise and following your doctor's orders, can help lower elevated cholesterol levels.

Today's Date

Take rest.
A field that has rested gives a beautiful crop.
—OVID

_____

Today's Date

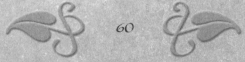

Avoiding caffeinated beverages, heavy meals,
and sugary snacks before bedtime can
help you get a better night's sleep.

Today's Date

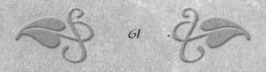

> The brain grows to the exact
> modes in which it has been exercised.
>
> —WILLIAM JAMES

Today's Date

Logic problems, crossword puzzles, cryptograms, and other mindbenders can provide your brain with a good workout.

Today's Date

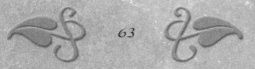

> The greatest of follies is to
> sacrifice health for any other kind of happiness.
> —ARTHUR SCHOPENHAUER

Today's Date

If you're a smoker, speak to your doctor about trying one of the many smoking-cessation aids available to you. Determination is a key to successfully quitting.

Today's Date

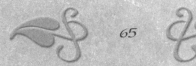

The ingredients of health and
long life are great temperance, open air,
easy labor, and little care.
—SIR PHILIP SIDNEY

_____

Today's Date

Common indoor plants such as golden pothos, peace lily, and ficus can help improve the air quality in your home or office.

Today's Date

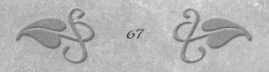

> The preservation of health is a duty.
> Few seem conscious that there is such a thing
> as physical morality.
>
> —HERBERT SPENCER

Today's Date

_____

_____

_____

_____

_____

_____

_____

_____

_____

_____

_____

_____

_____

_____

_____

_____

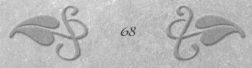

Infectious bacteria live in raw foods. Before, during, and after preparing foods—especially beef, pork, poultry, and fish—disinfect countertops and other surfaces, as well as any utensils used.

_____

Today's Date

> A crust eaten in peace
> is better than a banquet partaken in anxiety.
>
> —AESOP

Today's Date

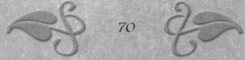

Proper digestion of the foods you eat is essential to good health. Chewing your food thoroughly is an important first step in this process.

Today's Date

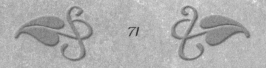

The sense of humor is the oil of
life's engine. Without it, the machinery creaks and
groans. No lot is so hard, no aspect of things is so grim,
but it relaxes before a hearty laugh.

—GEORGE S. MERRIAM

Today's Date

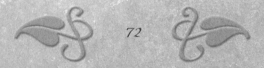

Hearty laughter is a wonderful stress reliever.
Foster a good sense of humor by partaking often
in whatever it is that gets you giggling.

Today's Date

The sovereign invigorator of the body is exercise,
and of all the exercises walking is the best.

— THOMAS JEFFERSON

Today's Date

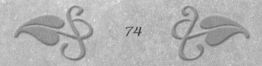

To stay fit, start and end your day with a brisk fifteen-minute walk. Walking promotes the circulation of blood throughout the body and generates an overall feeling of well-being.

Today's Date

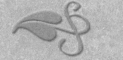

> Rest, as soon as there is pain,
> is a great restorative in all disturbances of the body.
>
> —HIPPOCRATES

Today's Date

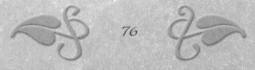

Getting seven to eight hours of sleep each night can help you function better throughout the day and can improve your general health.

Today's Date

_____

_____

_____

_____

_____

_____

_____

_____

_____

_____

_____

_____

_____

_____

_____

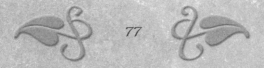

> Health is the first of all liberties,
> and happiness gives us the energy
> which is the basis of health.
> —HENRI FREDERIC AMIEL

_____

Today's Date

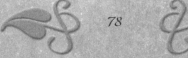

Before engaging in any new activity or exercise program, it's a good idea to undergo a complete physical examination and discuss your plans with your doctor.

Today's Date

> Things which matter most must never
> be at the mercy of things which matter least.
> —GOETHE

Today's Date

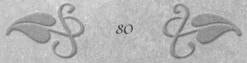

Managing your time can help reduce stress.
Set priorities and realistic goals,
but be sure to leave room for unexpected
diversions and downtime.

Today's Date

> # Time, Nature's great healer.
> —SENECA THE YOUNGER

Today's Date

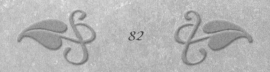

Acknowledging and expressing your grief is an important step toward coping with a loss or trauma and moving on with your life.

Today's Date

> Tell me what you eat,
> and I will tell you what you are.
>
> —ANTHELME BRILLAT-SAVARIN

_____

Today's Date

No single food, no matter how wholesome,
can provide your body with all of the
nutrients it needs to maintain good health.
Variety is the key to a healthy diet.

Today's Date

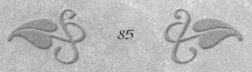

> Mind is the great lever of all things;
> human thought is the process by which human ends
> are ultimately answered.
>
> —DANIEL WEBSTER

Today's Date

Physical activity can help keep your mind sharp and alert by improving overall health and fighting stress and depression, both of which interfere with mental health.

Today's Date

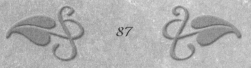

> To feel "fit as a fiddle"
> you must tone down your middle.
> —ANONYMOUS

Today's Date

Diets that promise rapid weight loss are seldom effective over the long term. Moreover, they often deprive the body of the necessary nutrients it needs to maintain health.

Today's Date

> Nothing is a waste of time
> if you use the experience wisely.
>
> —Auguste Rodin

Today's Date

Thoroughly wash vegetables and fruit
and remove the skin to reduce the chances of
ingesting pesticide or other chemical residue.

Today's Date

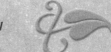

> True friendship is like sound health;
> the value of it is seldom known until it be lost.
> —CHARLES CALEB COLTON

Today's Date

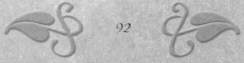

Avoid breathing in dangerous secondhand smoke. If you live with someone who smokes, ask your housemate to smoke outside.

Today's Date

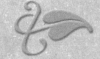

> Vigorous health and its
> accompanying high spirits are larger elements of
> happiness than any other things whatever.
>
> —HERBERT SPENCER

Today's Date

Paying close attention to your feelings and noting how you react to situations can help you recognize any irrational negative emotions that might be interfering with your happiness.

Today's Date

> Walking is the best possible exercise.
> Habituate yourself to walk very far.
>
> —THOMAS JEFFERSON

Today's Date

Whenever you're going to be outdoors for any length of time, be sure to apply sunblock to all exposed areas of your body no matter the weather or season.

_____

Today's Date

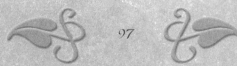

> What you can do, or dream you can, begin it;
> Boldness has genius, power and magic in it.
>
> —GOETHE

_____

Today's Date

A desire to make important lifestyle changes
is the first step toward leading a healthier life.
Confidence, commitment, and persistence
are the keys to success.

<u> </u>

Today's Date

> Worries go down better
> with soup than without.
>
> —JEWISH PROVERB

Today's Date

If you have a cold, go ahead and enjoy a bowl of chicken soup. Some studies suggest that it really does contain substances with medicinal properties.

_____

Today's Date

Youth is not a time of life—
it is a state of mind.

—ANONYMOUS

Today's Date

An animal companion, such as a dog or cat,
can help relieve loneliness, boredom,
and/or stress, among its many other
possible health benefits.

Today's Date

> Memory is the cabinet of the imagination, the treasury of reason, the registry of conscience, and the council chamber of thought.
>
> —GIAMBATTISTA BASILE

Today's Date

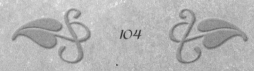

Brain-boosting supplements, such as phosphatidylserine (PS), ginkgo biloba, and DMAE, can help ward off cognitive decline and enhance mental function.

Today's Date

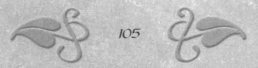

> Nothing great was ever
> achieved without enthusiasm.
>
> —RALPH WALDO EMERSON

Today's Date

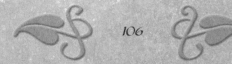

Fatigue can have many common causes, including lack of sleep, poor digestion, and stress. Herbal and nutritional supplements such as ginseng or CoQ_{10} can provide the body with a natural energy boost.

_____

Today's Date

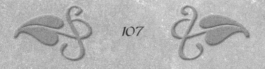

> A cluttered mind is
> little better than an empty one.
>
> —ANONYMOUS

Today's Date

Keep a calendar of scheduled activities and important dates. It can reduce the burden of having to remember too many things and help you avoid the guilt associated with forgetting.

Today's Date

A headache is a message
from the stomach to the brain saying,
"Don't send down any more garbage!"

—PHILIP YORDAN

Today's Date

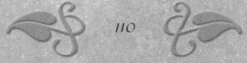

Recurrent or persistent headaches can sometimes be the result of a food allergy or intolerance. Eliminate suspect foods one at a time to see if this is the case.

Today's Date

> All gardeners live in beautiful places
> because they make them so.
>
> —JOSEPH JOUBERT

Today's Date

Gardening or yard work can be a good form of regular physical activity. In addition to a good workout, you may find that it also reduces stress and boosts your self-esteem.

Today's Date

An early morning walk
is a blessing for the whole day.
—HENRY DAVID THOREAU

Today's Date

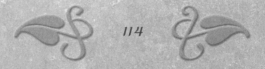

When choosing footwear, opt for comfort rather than style—especially if you are going to be on your feet all or most of the day.

Today's Date

> Beautiful young people are acts of nature,
> but beautiful old people are works of art.
> —ANONYMOUS

Today's Date

Glucosamine and chondroitin are among the natural products available that may help alleviate the pain of arthritis and slow down joint deterioration.

Today's Date

> Thought is the blossom;
> language the bud; action the fruit behind it.
>
> —Ralph Waldo Emerson

Today's Date

Infectious germs can be picked up from people, animals, and surfaces. Washing your hands often is one of the best ways to prevent the spread of infection.

Today's Date

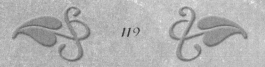

Carpe Diem! Rejoice while you are alive;
enjoy the day; live life to the fullest; make the most
of what you have. It is later than you think.

—HORACE

Today's Date

A positive mental attitude can get you over many hurdles in life. When people look only at the negative side of things, they bring themselves and others around them down.

_____

Today's Date

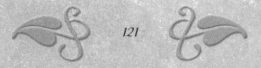

> Choose the life that is most useful,
> and habit will make it the most agreeable.
>
> —Francis Bacon

Today's Date

_____

_____

_____

_____

_____

_____

_____

_____

_____

_____

_____

_____

_____

_____

_____

_____

_____

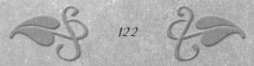

The quality and nutritional content of food is at its highest when the food is in season. An added benefit of seasonal foods is that an abundant supply keeps the cost low.

Today's Date

_____

> Don't let your sorrow
> come higher than your knees.
>
> —SWEDISH PROVERB

Today's Date

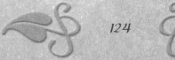

Swimming is an excellent form of exercise for people of all ages and activity levels. Among its many health benefits are improvements in strength and cardiovascular health.

Today's Date

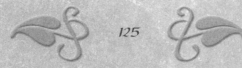

Your living is determined not so much by
what life brings to you as by what you bring to life.
—JOHN HOMER MILLER

Today's Date

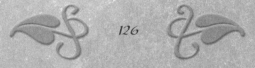

Food is best when fresh. Canned, frozen, overprocessed, and/or overcooked foods are lower in nutritional value, and some may even be completely lacking important nutrients.

Today's Date

_____

When you drink the water,
remember the spring.
—CHINESE PROVERB

Today's Date

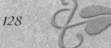

Try to drink six to eight 8-ounce glasses of pure water throughout the day, regardless of thirst, to keep your body properly hydrated.

Today's Date

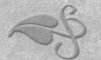
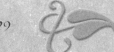

We are what we repeatedly do.
Excellence, then, is not an act, but a habit.

—ARISTOTLE

Today's Date

Coffee, soda, and other sugary beverages should not replace water in your diet. A lack of sufficient water can lead to disorders such as bad breath, constipation, and skin blemishes.

Today's Date

> Remedies often make diseases worse. . . .
> It takes a wise doctor to know when not to prescribe.
> —BALTASAR GRACIÁN

Today's Date

Antibiotics can deplete the healthy flora in the intestinal tract. Probiotic supplements such as acidophilus can help restore the balance.

Today's Date

Thousands of candles can be lighted from a
single candle, and the life of the candle will not be shortened.
Happiness never decreases by being shared.

—BUDDHA

Today's Date

When choosing candles for aromatherapy, avoid those made with synthetic fragrances. The packaging should indicate that "essential oils" were used in the product.

Today's Date

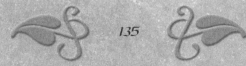

> There is no such thing
> in anyone's life as an unimportant day.
> —ALEXANDER WOOLLCOTT

Today's Date

It's a good idea to take time off from your daily workout routine to allow your muscles to recover and to give your body a chance to rest.

_____

Today's Date

> The real voyage of discovery consists not
> of seeking new landscapes, but in having new eyes.
> —MARCEL PROUST

Today's Date

Some things that happen in life may
be beyond your control. You can, however,
attempt to control your perception of events
by looking for a hidden lesson or purpose.

_____

Today's Date

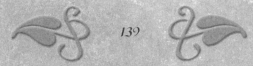

> Nothing will benefit human health
> and increase the chances for survival of life on Earth
> as much as the evolution to a vegetarian diet.
>
> —ALBERT EINSTEIN

_____

Today's Date

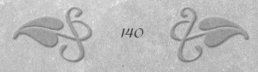

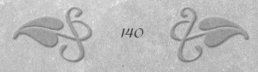

Those on a vegetarian or vegan diet must take extra steps to ensure that they are getting a healthy balance of all the nutrients the body needs—especially the essential amino acids, iron, and the B vitamins.

Today's Date

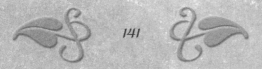

The freedom to make mistakes
provides the best environment for creativity.

—ANONYMOUS

Today's Date

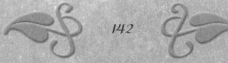

Compromised immunity is a liability. Keep your immune system strong with a good diet and by avoiding toxins. If you need a boost, immune-stimulating herbs such as echinacea may help.

Today's Date

> The more the mind receives,
> the more does it expand.
>
> —SENECA THE YOUNGER

Today's Date

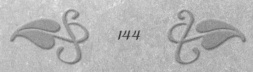

Active learning—for example, taking a class on a subject that interests you—can challenge your mind and keep your neurons firing.

Today's Date

> To conduct great matters and never
> commit a fault is above the force of human nature.
>
> —PLUTARCH

Today's Date

It is a mistake to ignore subtle clues that your health may be in jeopardy. Know the symptoms of serious illness and immediately report anything unusual to your doctor.

Today's Date

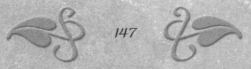

> We should manage our fortunes as we do our health—enjoy it when good, be patient when it is bad, and never apply violent remedies except in an extreme necessity.
>
> —FRANÇOIS LA ROCHEFOUCAULD

Today's Date

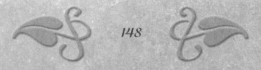

In matters of disease and treatments, it's wise to get a second opinion. In fact, many doctors expect their patients to do so before making any major decisions.

_____

Today's Date

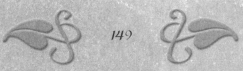

> To insure good health: Eat lightly,
> breathe deeply, live moderately, cultivate cheerfulness,
> and maintain an interest in life.
>
> —WILLIAM LONDEN

Today's Date

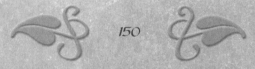

Try to leave yourself enough time during the day to enjoy a leisurely lunch or dinner with friends and/or family. Aim for at least one sit-down meal each day.

Today's Date

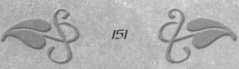

> What can anyone give you that is greater
> than this precious little instant known as "now"?
> —ANONYMOUS

_____

Today's Date

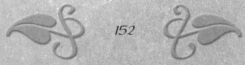

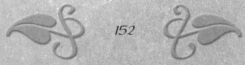

152

While it's a good idea to *plan* for the future, it's not such a good idea to *live* for the future. Too many sacrifices for a better tomorrow can detract from your appreciation of the present.

Today's Date

 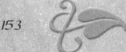

> Be aware of wonder. Live a balanced life—
> learn some and think some and draw and paint and sing
> and dance and play and work every day some.
> —ROBERT FULGHUM

Today's Date

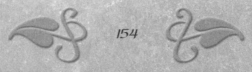

Art therapy is the therapeutic use of art-making under the guidance of a trained professional. It can help people overcome stress and traumas, increase self-awareness, and enhance cognition.

Today's Date

> When health is absent, wisdom cannot reveal itself,
> art cannot become manifest, strength cannot be exerted,
> wealth becomes useless, and reason is powerless.
>
> —HEROPHILUS

Today's Date

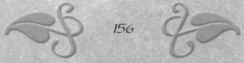

Controllable risk factors for heart disease include lack of exercise, smoking, poor diet, and high blood pressure. You *can* take steps to reduce your risk of this prevalent disease.

Today's Date

> A careful physician . . . before he attempts
> to administer a remedy to his patient, must investigate not
> only the malady of the man he wishes to cure, but also his habits
> when in health, and his physical constitution.
> —MARCUS TULLIUS CICERO

Today's Date

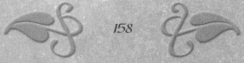

Holistic medicine blends traditional Western medicine with alternative or complementary therapies. Practitioners focus on treating the *whole* person: body, mind, and spirit.

Today's Date

> Our greatest weariness
> comes from work not done.
> —ERIC HOFFER

Today's Date

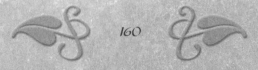

Putting off what needs to be done can negatively affect your outlook. Make an effort to stop procrastinating before the length of your to-do list exceeds the list of your accomplishments.

Today's Date

Aim at the sun, and you may not
reach it; but your arrow will fly higher than if aimed
at an object on a level with yourself.

—JOEL HAWES

Today's Date

Chronic conditions, such as diabetes, heart disease, and skin disorders, as well as some mental health illnesses, require ongoing healthcare management. This is best achieved by regularly scheduled doctor's visits.

> And silence, like a poultice, comes
> To heal the blows of sound.
>
> —OLIVER WENDELL HOLMES

Today's Date

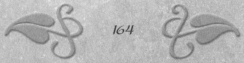

Food ingredients that may trigger migraine headaches include MSG, caffeine, and some artificial sweeteners. If you're prone to migraines, check product labels.

Today's Date

As we grow old, the beauty steals inward.

—BRONSON ALCOTT

Today's Date

Fall-related injuries are common among the elderly. To help prevent slips and falls in the home, remove tripping hazards, such as rugs and clutter, and improve lighting.

Today's Date

> Cultivate only the habits
> that you are willing should master you.
> —ELBERT HUBBARD

Today's Date

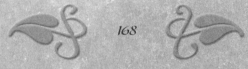

If you find yourself binging on unhealthy snacks, determine what triggers your binges and take steps to eliminate the trigger or learn to deal with it more effectively.

Today's Date

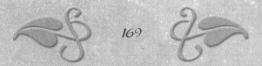

Character and conduct shape each other.

—ANONYMOUS

Today's Date

A healthy life begins with action—
accomplishing tasks, breaking addictions,
engaging in enjoyable activities, improving diet,
and getting adequate rest.

_____

Today's Date

_____

_____

_____

_____

_____

_____

_____

_____

_____

_____

_____

_____

_____

_____

_____

_____

_____

171

Better to strengthen your back
than lighten your burden.

—ANONYMOUS

Today's Date

To avoid back injury, don't bend at your waist to lift heavy items. Instead, squat down with your back straight, hold the item close to you, and stand up, letting your legs do the work.

Today's Date

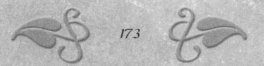

> Diet cures more than the lancet.
>
> —SPANISH SAYING

Today's Date

Vitamin C and vitamin E are two of the most powerful antioxidants and work in the body to protect your cells from harmful molecules known as free radicals.

Today's Date

> For fast-acting relief, try slowing down.
> —LILY TOMLIN

Today's Date

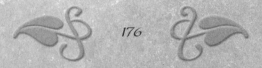

It's commonly known that a low calcium intake negatively effects bone health. What's not well known is that smoking and excessive use of alcohol can speed the rate of bone loss.

Today's Date

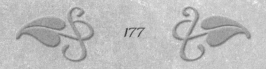

Plant your own garden and
decorate your own soul, instead of waiting for
someone to bring you flowers.

—VERONICA A. SHOFFSTALL

Today's Date

Bach Flower Remedies use oils extracted from flowers to heal negative emotions. Rescue Remedy—a combination of five different remedies—is a natural stress reliever.

_____

Today's Date

> Faith is not being sure
> where you're going but going anyway.
> —FREDERICK BUECHNER

_____

Today's Date

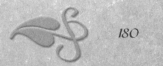

Research evidence suggests that religious involvement is associated with better physical and mental health. Studies are ongoing, as there is still much to be learned about the pathways by which religion affects health.

Today's Date

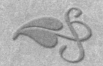

> The smile on your face is the light in
> the window that tells people that you are at home.
>
> —ANONYMOUS

Today's Date

To create a healthy home environment, ensure adequate ventilation. Open the windows often to let in fresh air. Also, keep surfaces clean and dry to prevent the growth of mold.

Today's Date

Earth laughs in flowers.
—RALPH WALDO EMERSON

_____

Today's Date

Drinking herbal tea is a pleasant way to derive the health benefits associated with herbs. When making tea, it's best to use fresh, pure water.

Today's Date

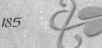

One should be just as careful in
choosing one's pleasures as in avoiding calamities.

—CHINESE PROVERB

_____

Today's Date

Protecting your health and the health of your family starts at home. Install smoke alarms and carbon monoxide detectors on every floor, and check batteries monthly.

Today's Date

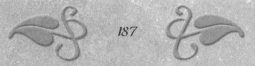

> Those who give cheerfully give twice—
> once to others, once to themselves.
>
> —ANONYMOUS

Today's Date

Healthy, supportive relationships can enhance your well-being and help you and loved ones through difficult times. Giving *and* receiving are essential to your involvement in a support system.

Today's Date

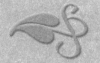
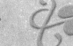

Dreams are renewable. No matter what our age
or condition, there are still untapped possibilities within us
and new beauty waiting to be born.

—DALE E. TURNER

Today's Date

Taking up a musical instrument you've always wanted to play or engaging in some other mentally challenging activity can help fend off mental deterioration.

Today's Date

> Destiny is not a matter of chance, it is
> a matter of choice; it is not a thing to be waited for,
> it is a thing to be achieved.
> —WILLIAM JENNINGS BRYAN

Today's Date

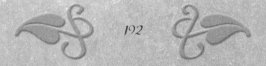

Retirees may find that traveling to new places can help them stay mentally and physically active. Planning these trips can also be stimulating and exciting.

_____

Today's Date

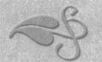

> Good friends are good for your health.
> —DR. IRWIN SARASON

Today's Date

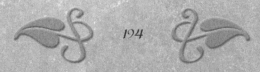

If you're a caretaker of an ailing loved one, consider joining a support group. Sharing your experiences with others may help make your task, and theirs, a little easier.

Today's Date

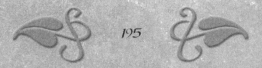

> ## Energy is Eternal Delight.
> —WILLIAM BLAKE

Today's Date

_____

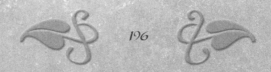

196

Among the many functions of the B vitamins are energy production and metabolism. As they are water-soluble, it's important to eat foods rich in the B vitamins or take supplements daily.

Today's Date

He who laughs, lasts!

—MARY PETTIBONE POOLE

Today's Date

Learning how to belly dance can be a fun way to get fit (and meet others). Belly dancing works muscles throughout the body and burns calories.

Today's Date

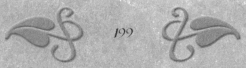

> Happiness is more a state of
> health than of wealth.
>
> —FRANK TYGER

Today's Date

If you are suffering from a migraine, try this for some immediate relief: Soak a towel in ice water, wring it out, then hold it against the back of your neck. Repeat as needed.

Today's Date

Home is where the heart is.

—PLINY THE YOUNGER

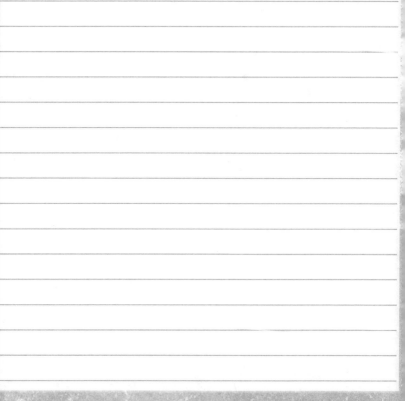

Today's Date

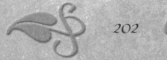

Have an escape plan from each room in
your house in case of a fire. Check windows
to be sure they open easily and make sure
you can reach the ground safely.

Today's Date

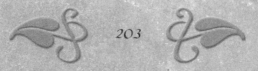

> If there is one single secret
> to long life, that secret is moderation.
>
> —GEORGE GALLOP

Today's Date

A proper balance of protein, fat, and carbohydrate is essential to good health. Include healthy sources of each of these macronutrients in your diet.

Today's Date

> The road to health is paved with
> vegetables, fruits, beans, rice and grains.
>
> —POLLY STRAND

Today's Date

_____

_____

_____

_____

_____

_____

_____

_____

_____

_____

_____

_____

_____

_____

_____

_____

Shop for fresh produce a few times a week so that you always have plenty of healthy food choices on hand for meals or snacks.

Today's Date

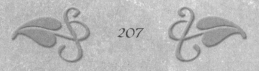

> # Failure teaches success.
> —JAPANESE SAYING

_____

Today's Date

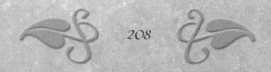

A headache is a warning signal from your body. While painkillers may provide short-term relief, it's important to determine and treat the underlying source of recurrent headaches.

_____

Today's Date

_____
_____
_____
_____
_____
_____
_____
_____
_____
_____
_____
_____
_____
_____
_____
_____
_____
_____

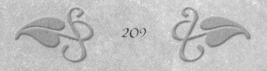

> If you wish to grow thinner,
> diminish your dinner.
>
> —HENRY SAMBROOKE LEIGH

Today's Date

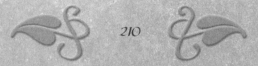

Learn the difference between "good" fats and "bad" fats, then eliminate or reduce the bad ones and up your consumption of the good ones.

Today's Date

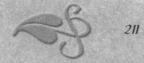

> It is remarkable how one's wits
> are sharpened by physical exercise.
> —PLINY THE YOUNGER

Today's Date

Staying physically fit without getting bored with your exercise program can be challenging. Consider your options to find a few different activities that will keep you interested.

_____

Today's Date

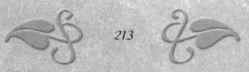

Learn to love good books. There are treasures in books that all the money of the world cannot buy, but that the poorest laborer can have for nothing.

—ROBERT G. INGERSOLL

Today's Date

It helps to stay informed regarding health and wellness. There are many helpful books that discuss specific health concerns or health and wellness in general.

Today's Date

A full Belly makes a dull Brain.

—BENJAMIN FRANKLIN

Today's Date

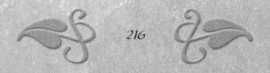

Peanuts are not actually nuts but legumes. However, just like nuts, they are high in protein, fiber, and unsaturated fats. They also contain an abundant supply of vitamins and minerals.

Today's Date

> A little nonsense now and then
> is cherished by the wisest men.
> —ROALD DAHL

Today's Date

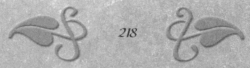

Some leisure activities can help keep you physically fit. For example, sports, gardening, and hiking can provide an enjoyable and rewarding whole-body workout.

Today's Date

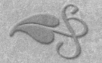

> A stumble may prevent a fall.
> —Thomas Fuller

_____

Today's Date

Avoid possible hazards when hiking.
For example, carry an adequate supply of water,
know how to recognize poisonous plants,
and always watch where you are stepping.

Today's Date

> Behold the turtle. He makes
> progress only when he sticks his neck out.
> —JAMES BRYANT CONANT

Today's Date

Acupressure is an ancient hands-on therapeutic technique that targets certain points on the body. It can help relieve pain associated with many health conditions.

Today's Date

Fall seven times, stand up eight.

—JAPANESE PROVERB

_____

Today's Date

_____

_____

_____

_____

_____

_____

_____

_____

_____

_____

_____

_____

_____

_____

_____

_____

_____

_____

Never use a piece of furniture in place of a ladder. This is a common fall hazard. When using a ladder, be sure to use it correctly and make sure it's stable.

Today's Date

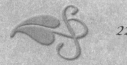

Every day is a once-in-a-lifetime day.

—ANONYMOUS

Today's Date

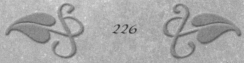

Taking your multivitamin and multimineral supplement along with a meal may increase your body's ability to absorb the nutrients.

Today's Date

He who would leap high
must take a long run.
—DANISH PROVERB

_____

Today's Date

Select shoes that are appropriate for your fitness activity and your particular needs. When choosing footwear for your sport, consult a knowledgeable salesperson.

Today's Date

> A journey of a thousand miles
> must begin with a single step.
> —CHINESE SAYING

Today's Date

When given a choice between riding an escalator or climbing stairs, opt for the stairs. Likewise, when parking, park further away for an invigorating walk to your destination.

Today's Date

Clearly, if disease is manmade, it can also be man-prevented. It should be the function of medicine to help people die young as late in life as possible.

—Dr. Ernst Wunder

Today's Date

An important key to maintaining good health is getting a yearly physical exam from your doctor. If you have a chronic health condition, more frequent checkups may be needed.

_____

Today's Date

> Faith is the strength by which
> a shattered world shall emerge into the light.
> —HELEN KELLER

Today's Date

Discuss the pros and cons of any medication you plan to take with your doctor or pharmacist to determine if the benefits outweigh the possible side effects.

Today's Date

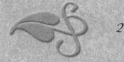

235

Let your food be your medicine,
and your medicine be your food.

—HIPPOCRATES

_____

Today's Date

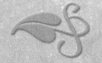

Almonds are high in protein, unsaturated fat, vitamin E, phosphorus, calcium, magnesium, and fiber. Eat almonds in moderation as part of a healthy diet.

Today's Date

A joyful heart makes a fair face.

—ANONYMOUS

Today's Date

Aerobic exercise can help keep your skin healthy. Sweating cleans the pores and triggers the production of sebum—the skin's own natural moisturizer.

_____

Today's Date

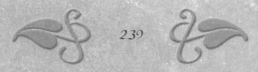

> It is always well to accept your own shortcomings with candor but to regard those of our friends with polite incredulity.
>
> —RUSSELL LYNES

Today's Date

Carrying around grudges can affect your happiness. To avoid resentment, share your feelings with anyone who has caused you hurt or anger in an effort to resolve the issue.

Today's Date

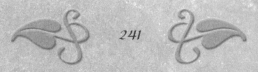

Keep changing.
When you're through changing, you're through.
—BRUCE BARTON

Today's Date

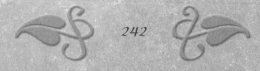

Change keeps things interesting and can prove beneficial to your health. Try to see change as an opportunity to expand your mind and your horizons.

Today's Date

> He that observeth the wind shall not sow;
> and he that regardeth the clouds shall not reap.
> —ECCLESIASTES 11:4

_____

Today's Date

To help you avoid dry skin, keep the air in your home from becoming too dry. Use a humidifier or place a bowl of water in each room. Plants help add moisture to the air, too.

Today's Date

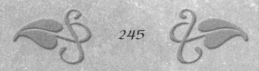

> Little strokes fell great oaks.
> —BENJAMIN FRANKLIN

Today's Date

People tend to underestimate the amount of calories they consume—especially when dining out. To avoid this, set aside a portion of your meal to take home and enjoy the next day.

Today's Date

> Life is what happens to you
> while you're busy making other plans.
>
> —JOHN LENNON

Today's Date

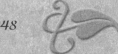

Many people who lead busy lives find it hard to fit exercise into their schedules. Ten minutes of moderate activity morning, noon, and evening should be possible for even the busiest person.

Today's Date

> You can't plant a seed
> and pick the fruit the next morning.
> —Reverend Jesse Jackson

_____

Today's Date

Here are some ways to include more fruit in your diet: top cereal with banana, toss berries into salads, blend peach slices into yogurt, and choose fruit salad over fattening dessert.

Today's Date

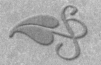

A merry heart doeth good like a medicine.
—OLD TESTAMENT

Today's Date

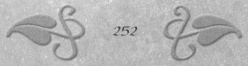

Insulin resistance, a condition in which the body does not use insulin properly, increases the risk of diabetes and heart disease. Possible causes include excess weight and too many refined carbohydrates.

Today's Date

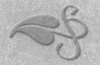

> To safeguard one's health at the cost
> of too strict a diet is a tiresome illness indeed.
>
> —FRANÇOIS LA ROCHEFOUCAULD

Today's Date

Calcium is not only vital for the formation of strong bones and teeth, but it also plays an essential role in various physiological functions, including muscle contraction.

Today's Date

> When fate hands us a lemon,
> let's try to make a lemonade.
> —DALE CARNEGIE

Today's Date

Citrus fruit such as oranges, lemons, and grapefruits are chockful of nutrients. They contain significant amounts of fiber and are rich in antioxidants and plant chemicals with health-promoting properties.

Today's Date

> We must always change, renew,
> rejuvenate ourselves; otherwise we harden.
>
> —GOETHE

Today's Date

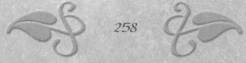

CoQ_{10} is a natural heart-protective nutrient. Although the body produces this substance, CoQ_{10} supplementation may offer some benefits against atherosclerosis and coronary artery disease.

Today's Date

After winter comes the summer.
After night comes the dawn. And after every storm,
there comes clear, open skies.

—SAMUEL RUTHERFORD

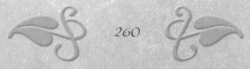

Seasonal affective disorder (SAD) is a mood disorder linked to a decrease in daylight during dark winter months. Talk to your doctor about how to avoid or reduce SAD before the winter blues hit.

Today's Date

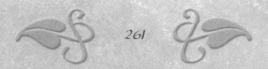

Cheerfulness is the best promoter of health
and is as friendly to the mind as to the body.
—JOSEPH ADDISON

_____
Today's Date

Aromatherapy is sometimes useful for relieving headache pain. For example, inhaling a blend of peppermint and lavender essential oils can provide relief. Consult a book on aromatherapy for blends to try.

Today's Date

> Bite off more than you can chew, Then chew it.
> Plan more than you can do, Then do it.
> —ANONYMOUS

_____

Today's Date

An aging body typically produces reduced amounts of stomach acid, interfering with the body's absorption of nutrients. This makes it especially important for older people to eat slowly and to chew their food thoroughly.

Today's Date

You can only cure retail
but you can prevent wholesale.
—BROCK CHISHOLM

Today's Date

Seat belts can help prevent serious injuries in a car accident. Whether you are a driver or a passenger, always wear your seat belt. A little discomfort is worth the benefits.

Today's Date

> When you cannot get a compliment
> any other way pay yourself one.
> —MARK TWAIN

Today's Date

People who *always* criticize you and your ideas
may cause you to question your own self-worth.
Make a list of supportive people in your life
and try to spend more time with them.

Today's Date

You better live your best and act your best and
think your best today, for today is the sure preparation for
tomorrow and all the other tomorrows that follow.

—HARRIET MARTINEAU

Today's Date

Preventive health care involves good habits, including exercise, weight control, proper nutrition, avoidance of toxins, periodic medical screenings, and recommended immunizations.

Today's Date

> There are only two ways to live your life.
> One is as though nothing is a miracle.
> The other is as if everything is.
> —ALBERT EINSTEIN

Today's Date

Bee products are known for their healing properties. For instance, bee pollen is loaded with nutrients and is associated with health benefits such as increased energy production and enhanced immunity.

Today's Date

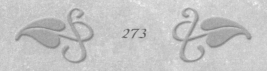

> Thou shouldst eat to live;
> not live to eat.
>
> —CICERO

Today's Date

Meats and whole-milk dairy products tend to be high in saturated fat. While some saturated fat may be necessary, a diet high in this type of fat has been linked to cardiovascular disease.

Today's Date

> All the art of living lies in
> a fine mingling of letting go and holding on.
> —HAVELOCK ELLIS

Today's Date

Letting go of negative emotions can improve
your overall health. If you feel negativity has
taken a stronghold, you may wish to work out
your feelings with the help of a counselor.

Today's Date

Enjoy present pleasures
in such a way as not to injure future ones.

—SENECA

_____

Today's Date

Although not every disease can be prevented, each time you make a healthy choice you are that much closer to a healthy future. Before engaging in harmful behavior, think about the consequences.

_____

Today's Date

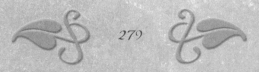

First say to yourself what you
would be; and then do what you have to do.

—EPICTETUS

Today's Date

id="1"

Having realistic goals can give you something
to strive for. When setting goals, it helps to be
as specific as possible. To make them easier to
achieve, break them down into small increments.

_____

Today's Date

_____

_____

_____

_____

_____

_____

_____

_____

_____

_____

_____

_____

_____

_____

_____

_____

> Grass is the hair of the earth.
> —Thomas Dekker

Today's Date

Wheatgrass juice—sometimes called a "superfood"—is a natural cleanser and detoxifier, and is rich in essential nutrients.

Today's Date

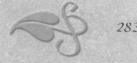

He that is of a merry heart
hath a continual feast.
—OLD TESTAMENT

Today's Date

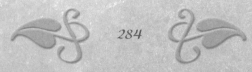

Resveratrol is a plant chemical with heart- and cancer-protective properties. It is found mainly in red wine and also in peanuts. These items should be consumed in moderation, so don't go overboard.

Today's Date

Moderation is medicine.

— BURMESE SAYING

Today's Date

It helps to pay attention to portion size to avoid overeating. For example, a three-ounce serving of beef, chicken, or fish is about the size of a deck of playing cards.

_____

Today's Date

Great thoughts come from the heart.

—MARQUIS OF VAUVENARGUES

Today's Date

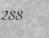

Taking care of your body can improve your outlook on life and enhance your mental health. Exercise, for example, may help alleviate depression, anxiety, and anger, as well as boost your self-esteem.

Today's Date

> Never argue at the dinner table,
> for the one who is not hungry always gets
> the best of the argument.
> —RICHARD WHATELY

Today's Date

Mealtimes should be enjoyed in a relaxed atmosphere. Waiting until after meals to discuss issues that may be upsetting will give you and your family uninterrupted time to take pleasure in, and derive the benefits of, your food.

_____

Today's Date

He who enjoys good health is rich,
though he knows it not.

—ITALIAN PROVERB

Today's Date

_____

_____

_____

_____

_____

_____

_____

_____

_____

_____

_____

_____

_____

_____

_____

_____

_____

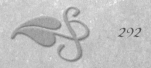

When thinking of what to give a loved one, how about givng a "gift of health"? For example, consider a set of dumbbells, a quality water bottle, a gift basket of healthy snacks, or a certificate to a fitness center.

_____

Today's Date

> Leisure does body and soul good.
> —GERMAN SAYING

Today's Date

Spend at least a half hour each day doing something that gives you pleasure, such as reading a good book, playing a game, working on a hobby, or talking to a friend.

Today's Date

Keeping your body healthy
is an expression of gratitude to the whole cosmos—
the trees, the clouds, everything.

—THICH NHAT HANH

Today's Date

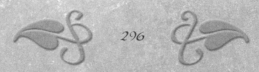

Proper breathing is important for vibrant health and energy. If you are a shallow breather, consider "retraining your breath" with breathing exercises a few times each day.

_____

Today's Date

> Good health and good sense
> are two of life's greatest blessings.
> —PUBLIUS SYRUS

Today's Date

Many people believe that coffee can sober them up after a bout of overdrinking. This is not true. Coffee cannot speed the time it takes for the liver to process alcohol.

Today's Date

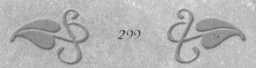

> As I see it every day you do one of two things:
> build health or produce disease in yourself.
>
> —ADELLE DAVIS

Today's Date

With the human brain being about 75 percent water, even moderate dehydration can cause dizziness and headaches. So be sure to drink several glasses of plain water throughout the day.

Today's Date

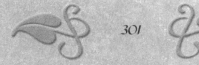

> Always behave like a duck—
> keep calm and unruffled on the surface
> but paddle like the devil underneath.
> —JACOB BRAUDE

Today's Date

In times of stress, inhaling the aroma of pure essential oils such as lavender and mandarin can produce a sense of calm and peacefulness.

Today's Date

> He who would live long
> must sometimes change his way of living.
>
> —ITALIAN SAYING

Today's Date

 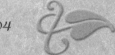

Carotenoids such as beta-carotene and lycopene are powerful antioxidants found in plants. They give fruits and vegetables their rich colors. If you don't eat a variety of fresh produce, try carotenoid supplements.

Today's Date

> Memory may be rendered duller
> or more retentive by the condition of the body.
> —QUINTILLIAN

_____

Today's Date

Some people unconsciously use alcohol or other drugs to "self-medicate" to relieve symptoms of a mental disorder. A mental health professional may help pinpoint the underlying reasons for the addiction.

Today's Date

> Meditate. Live purely. Be quiet.
> Do your work with mastery.
> Like the moon, come out from behind the clouds!
> Shine.
> —BUDDHA

Today's Date

_____

People of all faiths and walks of life meditate for various reasons. Among its many possible benefits, meditation helps relax the mind and body, which can lead to a more positive view of life.

Today's Date

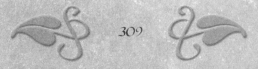

Luck is not chance—It's Toil—
Fortune's expensive smile is Earned—

—EMILY DICKINSON

_____

Today's Date

_____
_____
_____
_____
_____
_____
_____
_____
_____
_____
_____
_____
_____
_____
_____
_____
_____
_____
_____

Plaque buildup is the number-one cause of tooth decay and gum disease. Brush at least twice a day or after every meal and floss regularly. Have your teeth cleaned twice a year or more often if necessary.

Today's Date

> Don't tell your friends about your indigestion.
> "How are you" is a greeting, not a question.
> —ARTHUR GUITERMAN

Today's Date

Psyllium seeds and husks are rich in soluble fiber, which is important for digestive health. If you need more fiber in your diet, talk to your doctor about supplementing with psyllium.

Today's Date

Every sore has its salve.

—ENGLISH SAYING

Today's Date

Aloe vera is a well-known healing plant that aids tissue regeneration. It is often used to soothe and heal minor burns and wounds. As a houseplant, its healing properties can be kept close at hand.

Today's Date

315

> Seek the wisdom of the ages,
> but look at the world through the eyes of a child.
> —RON WILD

_____

Today's Date

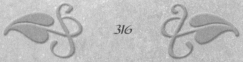

Children need a safe environment in which to grow and explore. If you have little ones, search your home from the eye level of a child for potential danger and remove it.

Today's Date

> Those who contemplate the beauty
> of the earth find reserves of strength that will
> endure as long as life lasts.
> —RACHEL CARSON

Today's Date

Performed properly, strength training can improve muscle mass and bone density, which can make you less prone to injuries. It can also speed up your metabolism, which reduces body fat.

_____

Today's Date

> What is required is sight and insight—
> then you might add one more: excite.
>
> —ROBERT FROST

_____

Today's Date

Even if you do not have vision problems, a yearly eye exam is an important part of health maintenance. Some eye diseases do not have symptoms but can be detected by an eye doctor.

Today's Date

> The pleasantest things in the world
> are pleasant thoughts: and the great art of life
> is to have as many of them as possible.
>
> —MONTAIGNE

Today's Date

When it comes to treating anxiety, there is a wide variety of natural products to choose from, including herbal supplements, teas, tinctures, essential oils, and homeopathic remedies.

Today's Date

The harder the nut,
the sweeter the kernel.

—Anonymous

Today's Date

Nuts contain mostly "good" fats, which can have a beneficial effect on heart health. They are also rich in other nutrients. Consider eating a handful of unsalted mixed nuts daily to derive their health benefits.

Today's Date

> You cannot turn back the clock.
> But you can wind it up again.
> —BONNIE PRUDDEN

Today's Date

Anti-aging medicine focuses on slowing down age-related biological processes. *The New Anti-Aging Revolution* by Drs. Klatz and Goldman is a good resource for anyone interested in this fast-growing field.

Today's Date

> The greatest strength
> and wealth is self-control.
>
> —PYTHAGORAS

_____

Today's Date

Rewarding yourself appropriately every time you avoid a negative habit can help reinforce your desire to stop. Identifying situations and feelings that trigger your habit can also help.

_____

Today's Date

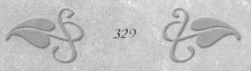

> The most important promises
> are the ones I make to myself.
>
> —MARY ANNE RADMACHER

Today's Date

People with allergies may find natural relief with the help of homeopathic remedies. Remedies target not only specific symptoms but also take into account certain other characteristics of health and behavior.

Today's Date

When we are tired,
we are attacked by ideas we conquered long ago.
—FRIEDRICH NIETZSCHE

Today's Date

You may find that fifteen minutes of meditation during the day can be as restful as a nap. Sit quietly with your eyes closed, be conscious of your breathing, and allow your thoughts to come and go.

Today's Date

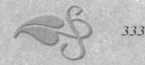

The secret of health for both mind
and body is not to mourn for the past, not to worry
about the future, or not to anticipate troubles, but to live the
present moment wisely and earnestly.

—BUDDHA

Today's Date

Some wild animals may have rabies—
a dangerous virus carried in the saliva of
an infected animal. Steer clear of all wildlife
and strays. In the case of a bite, seek
immediate medical attention.

Today's Date

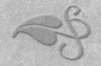

> The first wealth is health.
>
> —RALPH WALDO EMERSON

Today's Date

Use a piggy bank to keep track of your health. Each time you do something positive, deposit a dime; each time you do something unhealthy, withdraw a dime. If you run low on dimes, reconsider your actions.

Today's Date

> The greater danger for most of us
> is not that our aim is too high and we miss it.
> But that it is too low . . . and we reach it.
> —MICHELANGELO

Today's Date

Tea tree oil is an effective treatment for some cases of athlete's foot. For best results, it must be used consistently. Healing can be quickened when the oil is used along with complementary therapies.

Today's Date

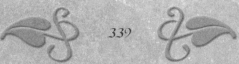

Sow a thought, reap an act;
Sow an act, reap a habit; Sow a habit, reap a character;
Sow a character, reap a destiny.
—ANONYMOUS

_____

Today's Date

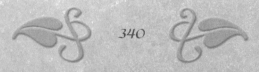

Hiccups usually pass relatively quickly with or without the help of common remedies. Recurrent, persistent hiccups, however, may indicate a condition that requires medical attention.

Today's Date

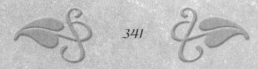

> Enthusiasm is the great hill-climber.
>
> —ELBERT HUBBARD

Today's Date

To protect yourself from prolonged exposure to the sun, keep an extra bottle of sunblock and a wide-brimmed hat in your car for unexpected outdoor excursions.

Today's Date

Health is not simply the absence of sickness.

—HANNAH GREEN

Today's Date

Poor oral health and hygiene can have serious health consequences. Take steps to maintain healthy teeth and gums and visit your dentist regularly.

Today's Date

> May you have enough happiness to make
> you sweet, enough trials to make you strong, enough sorrow
> to keep you human, enough hope to make you happy.
>
> —ANONYMOUS

Today's Date

For the freshest, most nutrient-rich juice,
consider juicing produce at home.
Remember, juicers remove most of the fiber,
so don't forego eating the whole fruit
or vegetable all of the time.

_____

Today's Date

> Ill-health, of body or of mind,
> is defeat. Health alone is victory. Let all men, if they
> can manage it, contrive to be healthy!
>
> —THOMAS CARLYLE

Today's Date

348

To reduce nausea during pregnancy, don't wait until mealtimes to eat. Rather, have many small meals throughout the day whenever hunger strikes. Also, choose bland foods over spicy or strong-smelling foods.

Today's Date

> Money is to my social existence
> what health is to my body.
> —MASON COOLEY

Today's Date

Associated with various health-promoting properties, green tea contains a higher concentration of nutrients than black tea. Green tea extract is available in supplement form.

Today's Date

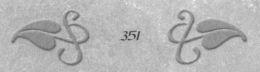

Life is not a "brief candle." It is a splendid torch that I want to make burn as brightly as possible before handing on to future generations.
—GEORGE BERNARD SHAW

Today's Date

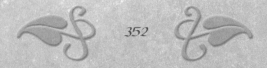

Normally produced by the pineal gland, melatonin is a hormone that regulates the body's internal clock. When traveling between time zones, the proper use of melatonin supplements may help relieve jet lag.

Today's Date

> Never underestimate your power
> to change yourself; never overestimate your
> power to change others.
> —H. JACKSON BROWN, JR.

Today's Date

Endorphins are natural mood-enhancing compounds produced by the body in response to stimulus such as exercise. Chances are if you are feeling down, you won't want to exercise, but it will surely improve your mood.

Today's Date

Man does not live by bread alone,
but he also does not live long without it.

—FREDERICK BUECHNER

Today's Date

Many popular processed foods and beverages contain high levels of sodium. This often results in consuming more of this mineral than the body needs. If this concerns you, check labels and go easy on the table salt.

Today's Date

One ought, every day at least, to hear
a little song, read a good poem, see a fine picture, and,
if it were possible, to speak a few reasonable words.

—GOETHE

_____

Today's Date

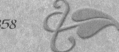

Repeated exposure to loud noise can lead to permanent hearing loss or ringing in the ears. Take steps to avoid hazardous noise or use hearing-protection devices.

Today's Date

> Hasty climbers have sudden falls.
> —JOHN CLARKE

_____

Today's Date

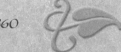

Taking a few bottles of water with you when you go out is a convenient way to make sure that you'll have plenty of opportunity to drink fresh water throughout the day.

Today's Date

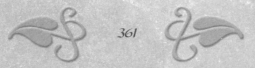

> Life was meant to be lived,
> and curiosity must be kept alive. One must never,
> for whatever reason, turn his back on life.
> —ELEANOR ROOSEVELT

Today's Date

While nosebleeds resulting from broken blood vessels can usually be treated at home, frequent or persistent nosebleeds can be a sign of trouble and should be brought to a doctor's attention.

Today's Date

No great thing is created suddenly,
any more than a bunch of grapes or a fig. If you tell me
that you desire a fig, I answer you that there must be time.
Let it first blossom, then bear fruit, then ripen.
—EPICTETUS

_____

Today's Date

Change takes time, so don't expect overnight
miracles. Instead, work toward your goals
with diligence and devotion and you
will eventually reap the rewards.

Today's Date

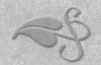

One cannot alter a condition with the same mind set that created it in the first place.
—ALBERT EINSTEIN

_____

Today's Date

Cranberry juice is a common remedy for urinary tract infections. When buying cranberry juice for this reason, opt for 100 percent juice with no added sugar.

Today's Date

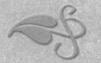
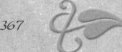

> If we could give every individual the right amount of nourishment and exercise, not too little and not too much, we would have found the safest way to health.
>
> —HIPPOCRATES

Today's Date

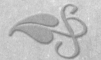
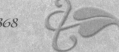

Each person has his or her own unique needs.
This is known as bioindividuality.
What works for one person may not work
for someone else. Discovering what's
right for you may take some time.

Today's Date

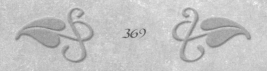

369

> Many hands make light work.
>
> —GREEK SAYING

Today's Date

When you're feeling overwhelmed by chores or work-related duties, asking others for assistance with specific tasks can help ward off tension and anxiety.

Today's Date

I find the medicine
worse than the malady.
—JOHN FLETCHER

_____

Today's Date

When considering taking a new medication (prescription or otherwise), learn as much as you can about it, including its proper use and possible side effects.

Today's Date

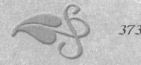

Memory . . . is the diary
that we all carry about with us.

—OSCAR WILDE

_____

Today's Date

Keeping a diary can help you recall special moments and important events in your life. Rereading what you have written at a later time can help keep those precious memories fresh and alive.

Today's Date

> Today is the first day
> of the rest of your life.
> —CHARLES DEDERICH

Today's Date

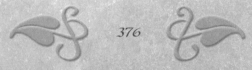

Yoga enhances one's ability to experience the interconnectedness of mind, body, and spirit. Regular practice can have a positive effect on various health conditions.

Today's Date

NOTES

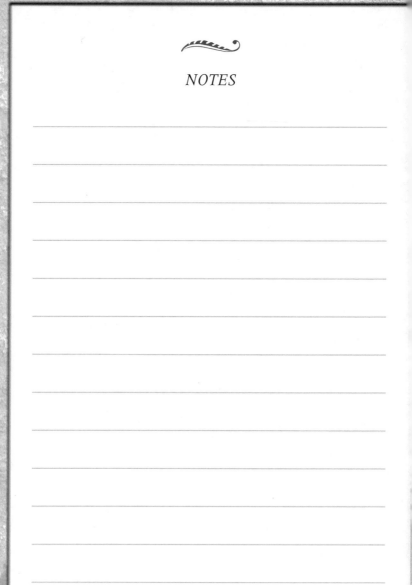

NOTES

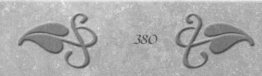

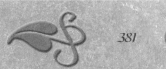